TREAT YOUR OWN BACK

Robin McKenzie was born in Auckland, New Zealand in 1931. He attended Wairarapa College and later graduated from the New Zealand School of Physiotherapy in 1952. After commencing private practise in Wellington in 1953, he developed a keen interest in the treatment of low back pain and subsequently attended the clinics of specialists in Europe and North America.

During the sixties, Mr McKenzie developed his own methods and since then has become recognised internationally as an authority on the treatment of low back pain. He has lectured in North America, Europe and Australasia where his methods for treating low back pain are now widely practised.

He is a member of the New Zealand Society of Physiotherapists, the New Zealand Manipulative Therapists Association, is a Consultant and Lecturer to the Orthopaedic Physical Therapy Programme at the Kaiser Permanente Medical Centre in Hayward, California, and is a Member of the Editorial Board for the North American Journal of Orthopaedic Physical Therapy and Sports Medicine.

Mr McKenzie has published two papers in the New Zealand Medical Journal, and he is the author of two books, "Treat Your Own Back", and "Mechanical Therapy and Diagnosis of the Lumbar Spine."

Treat your own back

*How to safely, simply
and scientifically
relieve your own
back pain*

by
ROBIN McKENZIE M.N.Z.S.P., M.N.Z.M.T.A.

Spinal Publications

Spinal Publications
Postal address: P.O. Box 2, Waikanae, New Zealand

© Robin McKenzie 1980

ISBN 0-473-00065-2

First Published in 1980
Second Edition   January, 1981
Reprinted   July, 1981
Reprinted   September, 1981
Reprinted   April, 1982
Reprinted   November, 1982
Reprinted   October, 1983
Reprinted   February, 1984

Printed by Wright and Carman Limited
Nicolaus Street, Upper Hutt
New Zealand

CONTENTS

INTRODUCTION

Low back pain is one of the most common ailments, for it affects nearly every one of us at some stage of our active adult life. It is described in many ways, such as slipped disc, lumbago, arthritis in the back, and ricked back.

When in acute pain we are usually unable to think clearly about our trouble, and simply seek relief from the pain. On the other hand, when we are recovered from an acute episode most of us quickly forget our low back problems.

Indeed, low back pain remains a mystery to most people: it often starts without warning and for no obvious reason; it interferes with simple activities of living, moving about, and getting a comfortable night's sleep, and then, just as unexpectedly, the pain subsides.

The causes of low back pain are no mystery. First, I will explain why low back pain may occur. Then I will suggest how you can avoid it; or, if at present you are having low back pain, how you may recover from it and prevent it from recurring.

The main point of this book is that the management of your back is *your* responsibility. Of course, you can call on people with particular skills for help — doctors and physiotherapists — but in the end only *you* can really help yourself. Self-treatment of low back pain is now widely accepted; it will be more effective in the long-term management of your low-back problems than any other form of treatment.

Many publications set out to tell you how to look after your own back, and you may well wonder why another is now offered. The reason is that this is the first book to show you how to 'put your back in', — to use the lay term —, if you are unfortunate enough to have 'put it out'; and, in addition, it shows you how to prevent your back from 'going out' again, once you have successfully 'put it back in'.

This book is not for you if you have developed low back pain for the first time; in that case you should consult your doctor, who will probably refer you to a manipulative therapist — a specialist physiotherapist — for treatment and, more important, for advice and instructions on the prevention of further low back problems.

You should also seek advice if there are complications to your low back pain; for example, if your trunk is pulled off-center, if you have muscle spasms, or severe and stabbing pains.

Finally, this book will help only eighty percent of people with low back pain; it is for those with straight-forward problems. I hope you prove to be amongst this eighty percent, and that you find the information clear and helpful.

R. McK.
Wellington
1980

1

LOW BACK PAIN

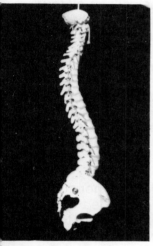

Photo 1
A head at the top
of this column
would be in profile,
facing right.

THE SPINE
Let us look at the human backbone (photo 1) — the spine or spinal column. This consists of the bones of the spine — the vertebrae —, and the cartilages in between them — the discs.

Each vertebra has a solid part in front (the body) and a hole in the back. When these holes are lined up as in the spinal column, they form a protected passageway (the spinal canal) which carries a bundle of nerves (the spinal cord) from head to pelvis.

Between each vertebra there is a small opening on either side, through which a nerve leaves the spinal cord — the right and left spinal nerve. This happens all along the spine so that there are thirty-one pairs of spinal nerves.

Among other tasks, the spinal nerves supply all the muscles in our body with the necessary energy to contract; and they tell us what we feel — things like hot and cold, pressure, and pain. In the lower part of the spine some of these nerves combine on each side to form the right and left sciatic nerves, which service our legs.

The discs are located between the bones of the vertebrae just in front of the spinal cord. Each disc can alter its shape, like a rubber washer, and this allows the spine to move in so many directions. However, when a disc distorts and protrudes backwards it may press painfully on the spinal cord or pinch a spinal nerve. Thus, in the low back, a 'slipped disc' — to use the lay term — may cause

3

low back pain and/or leg pain — sciatica — and sometimes other symptoms as well.

FUNCTIONS OF THE SPINAL COLUMN

The spinal column bears the weight of the top half of the body, transfers it to the pelvis, and from there to the seat (when sitting) or the feet (when standing, walking and running). Animals that walk on all fours do not have such an arrangement; the weight of the front part of their body is taken by their front legs, and that of the back part by their rear legs.

The main functions of the spinal column of four footed animals are to provide a strong flexible connection between the front and back of their body; and, particularly, to carry nerves in the protected passageway through the vertebrae. The spine of the upright human animal has those functions too, and the added function of bearing weight.

In the evolution from the four-legged horizontal-spine position of animals to the two-legged upright posture of man, the soft discs between the vertebrae have adapted to support heavier weights; and, more important, the spine has taken on a series of curves that ingeniously allow for better shock absorption and flexibility.

An engineer looking at a human skeleton would predict that most strains in the structure would occur in that area of the spine that is just above its junction with the pelvis. He would be right: this is where back problems usually arise: in the small of the back.

4

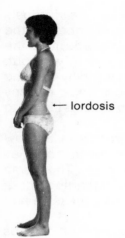

← lordosis

Photo 2

THE LORDOSIS — THE HOLLOW IN THE LOW BACK

The side view of the human body (photo 2) shows that there is a strong inward curve in the small of the back just above the pelvis. This hollow in the low back is the *lordosis*. It is the main curve in the spine that concerns us in this book.

When standing upright the lordosis is naturally present, though it varies from person to person. The lordosis is lost whenever the low back is rounded, and this usually occurs during sitting and bending. If the lordosis is lost often and for long enough periods, low back problems may develop.

WHY LOW BACK PAIN?

Mechanical pain occurs when the joint between two bones has been placed in a position that overstretches the surrounding tissues. This is true for mechanical pain in any joint — elbow, ankle or fingers for example — but in the spine there are additional factors: the tissues around the joints between vertebrae are also the retaining walls for the soft discs that act as a cushion between these same vertebrae. If the tissues around the discs are overstretched, the discs will distort and this may cause further pain. Then, to make matters worse, the distorted discs will prevent the vertebrae from lining up properly during movement, and this will further stretch other tissues around the discs and increase pain.

Many people think that low back pain is caused by 'strained muscles'. This is seldom the case. The cause of nearly all simple mechanical low back pain lies in the discs between the vertebrae, and in the tissues surrounding them.

Low back pain is frequently brought on by: sitting for a long time in a poor position (photo 3); prolonged bending (photo 4); heavy lifting (photo 5); bad working positions (photos 6, 7 and 8); and standing or lying for a long time in a poor position. When you look carefully at these photos you will see

5

that the low back is rounded — and *the lordosis has been lost.*

Unfortunately, many people lose the lordosis much of the time, and seldom (or never) increase the lordosis to its very maximum. People who lose the lordosis for long periods at a time, year in year out, and never properly restore it, will eventually lose the ability to keep a hollow in the low back for any length of time. These people are most likely to develop low back problems.

Most people naturally have a lordosis in the low back when they walk or run, and these activities often help in relieving low back pain. The same applies to standing, though when standing for a long time the lordosis often becomes excessive and may produce pain.

It follows that people with sedentary office jobs may easily develop low back pain. They often sit with a rounded back for hours on end (photo 8), and find that when they finally get up, the must walk stooped for a few yards before they can fully straighten up. The reason for this is that it takes a few minutes for the joints to recover from overstretching. *If this happens to you, and occurs often enough, you can expect low back pain to develop.* You must try to prevent this by sitting correctly with a good inward curve in your low back, and by regularly interrupting your sitting. How to do this will later be discussed in more detail (pages 24 and 25).

If a sedentary worker has acute or agonising low back pain when he stands up after prolonged sitting, it is almost certain that he has been sitting badly. This slouching has led to so much distortion in the discs that they cannot regain their proper shape quickly enough to allow normal movement. When movement is attempted the distorted discs stretch the surrounding tissues and produce pain. In addition, they may pinch nerves and cause other symptoms as well.

To stress the point again: *low back pain is likely to develop in the six situations shown (photos 3 to 8) because, in each, the lordosis has been lost.* The

6

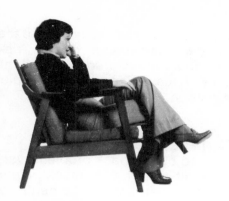

Photo 3

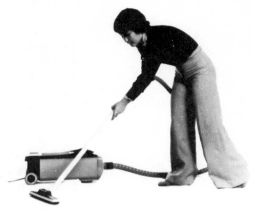

Photo 4

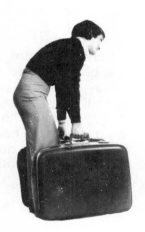

Photo 5

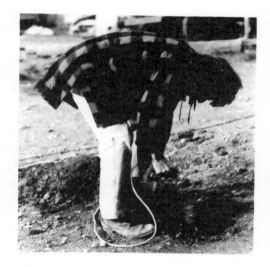

Photo 6

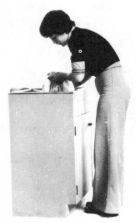

Photo 7

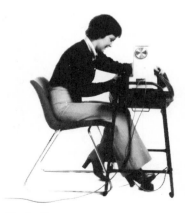

Photo 8

theme of this book is that pain can be avoided if the lordosis is *maintained,* especially during risk situations; or if it is *regularly restored* in situations where it cannot easily be maintained — for example, while weeding the garden.

WHERE IS THE PAIN FELT?

The sites of pain caused by low back problems vary from one person to another. In a first attack pain is usually felt at or near the belt line, in the center of the back (photo 9) or just to one side (photo 10), and it usually subsides within a few days.

In ·subsequent attacks pain may extend to the buttock (photo 11); and later still to the outside or back of the thigh down to the knee (photos 12 and 13), or below the knee down to the ankle or foot (photo 14).

Pain may vary with movement or with the position taken: the intensity of pain can change; or the site of pain can alter — for example, one movement may cause buttock pain, another may cause the pain to leave the buttock and appear in the low back.

If you have symptoms in the leg below the knee (photo 14) — for example, pain, pins and needles, numbness or weakness — it is likely that a nerve is being compressed in the low back. This could be serious ánd you should consult your doctor immediately.

WHO CAN PERFORM SELF TREATMENT?

To decide whether you can treat your own low back pain you must answer the following questions:
* Are there any periods in the day when you have no pain? Even ten minutes?
* Are you usually worse when sitting for prolonged periods or on arising from sitting?
* Are you usually worse during prolonged bending or stooping (as in bed making, vacuuming, ironing, gardening, concreting)?
* Are you often worse first thing in the morning, but improve after about half an hour?

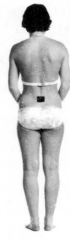
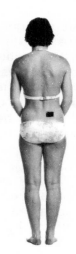
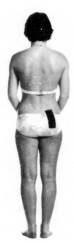

Photo 9   Photo 10   Photo 11

The black patch or line shows where pain may be felt.

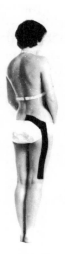
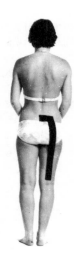
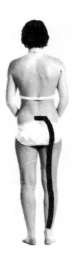

Photo 12   Photo 13   Photo 14

9

* Are you generally worse when inactive and better when on the move?
* Are you generally better when walking?
* Are you generally better when lying face down? (When testing this you may feel worse for the first few minutes after which time the pain subsides; in this case the answer to the question is 'yes').
* Is the pain confined to areas above your knee?
* Have you had several episodes of low back pain over the past months and years?

If you have answered 'yes' to all the questions you are an ideal subject for the self-treatment suggested in this book.

If you have answered 'yes' to any four or more questions your chances of benefit from the self-treatment are good and you should follow the programme.

If you have answered 'yes' to only three or fewer of the questions you should consult a manipulative therapist as some form of specialised treatment or manipulation may be necessary for you. This does not mean that the procedures recommended in this book will not apply to you in time; but at present the distortion in the affected joint is too great to be effectively reduced by the self help exercises. Once the severe pains have passed the exercise programme should be started. The exercises must be followed carefully.

2

RISK SITUATIONS

1. SITTING FOR PROLONGED PERIODS
This applies as much to people going on a long car journey, as to those sitting in office chairs at work or in lounge chairs watching television. To prevent low back pain you must (1) sit correctly, and (2) interrupt prolonged sitting at regular intervals ... stand up, stretch, ideally give yourself some exercise 4's.

Correct sitting
Bad sitting postures in themselves may *cause* low back pain. If you already have low back pain a poor slouched sitting posture will *prolong* low back pain and prevent rapid and complete recovery.

Regardless of the effects of Exercises 1 to 4 on the pain, you should pay a lot of attention to your sitting posture. You may have been sitting slouched for many years without back pain, but now that you have a 'bad back' you must no longer sit in the old way, because *this will only perpetuate the overstretching* discussed in the beginning of the booklet under WHY LOW BACK PAIN (page 5).

To sit correctly you must be fully practised in Exercise 5. The rhythmic 'slouch-overcorrect' procedure restores the lordosis; and the ten percent release of the extreme of the lordosis allows you to sit correctly indefinitely when on a seat without a back rest.

A lumbar supportive roll is essential. The principles of correct sitting must also be applied when sitting on a seat with a back rest. If you do not use a roll to *support the lordosis,* you will slouch as soon as you relax, or concentrate on anything other than holding the lordosis actively with your own muscles. You will slouch, for example, when talking, reading, writing, watching television, driving your car. To counteract this you must put a *supportive roll in the small of your back* when sitting in your easy chair (photos. 15 — wrong, and 16 — correct), office chair (photos. 17 — wrong, and 18 — correct), and car seat.

Lumbar roll

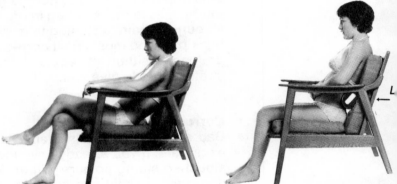

Photo 15: Bad.

Photo 16: Good.

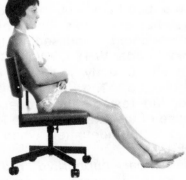

Photo 17: Bad.

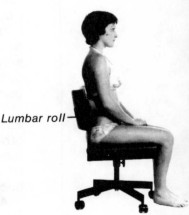

Lumbar roll

Photo 18: Good.

12

The roll should be no more than three to four inches in diameter before being compressed, and should be moderately filled with foam. The purpose of the roll is to hold your low back in a good but not extreme lordosis without you having to concentrate on it. The use of the roll may initially cause an increase in pain, brought about by maintaining a new position. This is normal and should wear off in a few days.

You can see a roll (end on) in photo 16. For this purpose a cushion will not do — it is the wrong shape.

Once you have become used to the correct way of sitting you will enjoy it. You will automatically choose chairs that allow you to sit properly — using a lumbar support when appropriate — and avoid those horrors that force you to sit slouched with a rounded back.

When you have been completely painfree for some weeks you may occasionally sit slouched, provided this is not maintained for too long and is always followed by some time spent in the corrected lordotic position to compensate for the distortion that may have occurred in the joints of your low back.

RULE: when sitting for prolonged periods you must sit correctly with the low back in lordosis, and use a lumbar support where the seat has a back rest.

Regular interruption of prolonged sitting.
Research has shown that even when you sit correctly with a good lordosis, the pressure within your discs is raised. When this increased pressure is present for long periods at a time, some distortion will take place in the joints containing the discs. Nearly everybody will be aware of some stiffness and discomfort in the low back after an uninterrupted car ride of some hours. If you already have back problems such a journey will make them much worse. Therefore, regular interruption of prolonged sitting is necessary to reduce the

pressures within the discs, and relieve the stresses on the surrounding tissues.

RULE: regular interruption of prolonged sitting is essential. This can be achieved by standing up, bending backwards five or six times, and walking about for a few minutes. These simple measures will usually prevent distortion in the joints of the low back so that pain will not occur.

If you are a desk worker you must make sure that your desk is the correct height, allowing your feet to be flat on the floor and your thighs to be horizontal and not pressing on the seat of the chair. The surface of the desk must be at the correct height as well, because if the surface you lean on is too low you will slouch forward and lose your lordosis. The chair should be pulled into the desk so that your stomach is gently held against the front of it, as this will prevent you from leaning over and losing the lordosis when writing or reading. The back of the chair should allow you to maintain a lordosis, and insert a lumbar support as you sit.

2. WORKING IN STOOPED POSITIONS
Many activities cause people to stoop: bench work, hobbies, sport, housekeeping, looking after small children, and so on.

Once you have had problems with your low back, and especially if these were caused by working in a stooped or bent position, you must become fully practised in Exercise 4 — backward bending in standing. When performed regularly this exercise will correct any distortion that tends to develop while working bent over or stooped; and when it is done *before pain starts* it will usually prevent significant low back pain.

If the regular performance of Exercise 4 has failed to prevent the onset of pain, you must immediately start with Exercise 3 — press-ups —, and if necessary repeat it many times.

RULE: While you are performing tasks which eliminate the lordosis, you must restore it at regular intervals. You may have to stand upright and bend backwards five or six times every ten minutes to prevent the onset of pain.

3. RELAXING AFTER VIGOROUS ACTIVITY

When you have finished some vigorous activity — for example, gardening or concreting — and have not suffered any pain as a result, *do not* relax by sitting slouched in a chair. Thoroughly exercised joints of the low back easily distort if they are held in the slouched position.

A commonly heard story is from the person who sits down to rest after vigorous activity, and some time later has excruciating pain which transfixes him so that he can hardly move at all. Most people blame the vigorous activity as the cause of the trouble; it is not usually so and in most cases the pain is produced by slouched relaxed sitting.

RULE: After vigorous activity you should keep the lordosis by backward bending in standing and/or press-ups. If you sit down to rest, do not slouch.

4. LIFTING

In order to avoid low-back strain when lifting, it is important that you lift correctly: accentuate the hollow in your back, bend your knees; hold the load close to you, lift by straightening your legs, and lean backwards to stay in balance (photo 19). After some practise at this you will automatically make a good lordosis and bend your knees properly before lifting.

If you are suffering a bout of low back pain it is best to completely avoid lifting for the time being; if this is not possible you must use the correct lifting

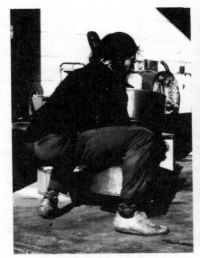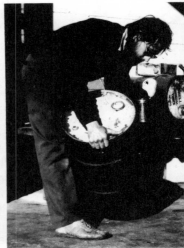

Photo 19: Good.   Photo 20: Bad.

technique and avoid at all times objects that are awkward to handle or heavier than thirty pounds. If you have no low back problems and have not been in a stooped or sitting position for some time before lifting, you may lift weights of up to thirty pounds without taking special care. *Under all other circumstances* you must be very careful and use the correct lifting technique.

Once you have low back problems you should never again handle awkward or heavy objects by yourself, even though you may be completely painfree at the time of lifting.

In order to minimise the risks involved in lifting you should always perform Exercise 4 — backward bending in standing — before and immediately after lifting; and if there are many objects to be lifted you must frequently interrupt the lifting and perform Exercise 4. If Exercise 4 is done before lifting it minimises the distortion present in the joints while you lift; if done after lifting it corrects any distortion that may have developed as a result of the lift.

RULE: To lift a weight you should squat as low as possible by bending the knees and keeping the back straight (vertical — see photo 19); lift by straightening the knees, still keeping the back straight. Absolutely avoid bending down and lifting with your back rounded and your legs straight (photo 20) for this can easily cause a sudden attack of low back pain.

Prolonged standing

Some people always get low back pain when standing in one place for a long time. This is because in relaxed standing their low back hangs in the extreme position with an excessive lordosis (photo 21).

If your low back pain comes on during prolonged standing you will find relief by actually reducing the lordosis. This is achieved by standing tall, lifting the chest up, pulling in the stomach muscles, and tightening the buttock muscles (photo 22). With some practise you can learn to stand in this new position for long periods without discomfort.

Lying

Although lying is not a risky situation, it still requires some discussion. Many people have low back pain when they are lying down, and some of these have pain *only when lying*. When the pain interferes with sleeping, people may gradually become irritable and unpleasant to live with.

If you have pain when lying down, you are placing strains on your low back in the lying position. There are several ways of arranging your bed that might reduce these strains.

The first way is to lie on a firm support that does not sag. Therefore you should avoid a wire base and use a solid base instead with a rubber or inner-spring mattress on top of it (photo 23).

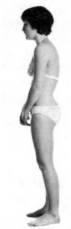 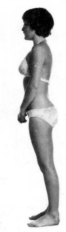

Photo 21
Slouched standing

Photo 22
Correct standing

If this brings no improvement within a week to your comfort at night, you should see if lying with a supportive roll around your waist brings relief. When you lie on your side the roll will fill the natural hollow in the body contour between pelvis and rib cage; and when you lie on your back the roll will support the lordosis. By folding a beach towel in half from end to end and rolling it from the side, you will

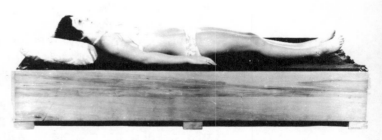

Photo 23: A firm base can have a thick mattress on it.

create a roll of about three to four inches across and three feet in length. Wind the roll around your waist, and fix it in front with a safety pin to ensure that it remains in place where you would normally wear your belt (if it moves up or down it may actually increase your night pain). When using the roll in bed your low back will be supported whether you are lying on your back or on either side (photos 24 — not supported, and 25 — supported).

If you have tried these suggestions, without benefit, you should consult a manipulative therapist. You may require specialist advice or manipulative treatment.

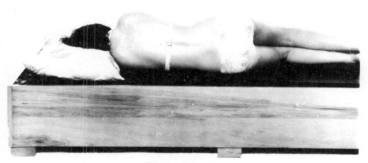

Photo 24

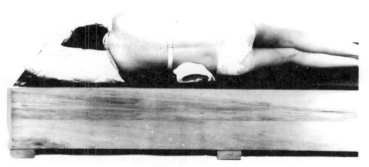

Photo 25

HIGH-RISK SITUATIONS

1. *Travelling long distances by car* without regular breaks which permit movement away from the sitting position. Advice: sit with a lumbar support, and at regular intervals and *before pain starts* get out of the car, bend backwards five or six times, and walk around for a few minutes. For some people it is enough to do this every two hours, though others will need to do it more often.

2. *Removing heavy objects from the boot — or trunk — of the car* immediately after driving. Advice: walk around for a few minutes and bend backwards five or six times before pulling out those heavy suitcases, then stand upright and bend backwards five or six times after lifting.

3. *Travel by plane,* when you may sit for a long time in a cramped seat. Advice: sit with a lumbar support; get up, bend backwards five or six times, and walk about in the plane at regular intervals. Visit the toilet whether you need to or not.

4. When working in stooped positions or lifting heavy and awkward objects especially *in the first four hours of the day* you are more liable to 'put your back out'. Advice: Frequently interrupt prolonged bending by standing upright and bending backwards five or six times; and before and after lifting you must also stand upright and bend backwards five or six times.

5. *Coughing and sneezing* when you are bent forwards or sitting. This may cause a sudden attack of low back pain or aggravate existing back pain. Advice: when you have low back problems you must try to stand up and bend backwards while coughing and sneezing. At least lean back and make the best lordosis you can.

3

EXERCISES

EXERCISE 1
Lie face down with your arms beside your body and
your head turned to one side (photo 26). Stay in this
position for about five minutes, making sure that you
relax completely.

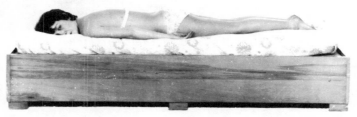

Photo 26: Exercise 1.

EXERCISE 2
Remain face down, but now lean on your elbows
(photo 27). Stay in this position for about five
minutes, making sure that you relax your low back
completely.

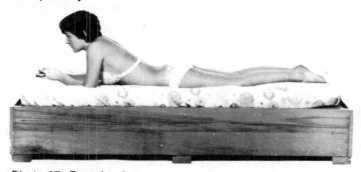

Photo 27: Exercise 2.

21

EXERCISE 3

Remain face down, but now place your hands in position for 'press-ups' (photo 28); press the top half of your body up as far as pain permits (photo 29), remembering at the same time to keep pelvis and legs hanging limp and to sag in the low back; then lower yourself to the starting position; repeat the exercise, moving higher each time *so that in the end you are as high as possible* with your arms as straight as possible (photo 30). You must repeat the exercise ten times per session, and spread the sessions evenly six to eight times throughout the day.

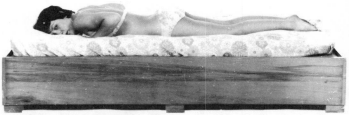

Photo 28: Exercise 3 "press-ups".

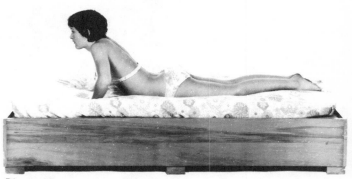

Photo 29

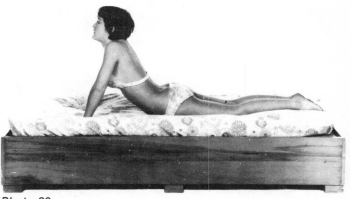

Photo 30

22

EXERCISE 4

Stand upright and place your hands in the small of your back (photo 31); bend backwards at your waist, using your hands as a fulcrum and keeping the knees as straight as possible (photo 32); then return to the upright standing position. When used in the *treatment* of low back pain the exercise should be repeated ten times per session, and the sessions should be spread evenly six to eight times throughout the day. When used as a *prevention* of low back pain the exercise should be repeated five or six times and should be performed as often as required.

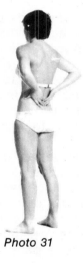

Photo 31

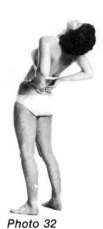

Photo 32

Exercise 4: Backwards bending.

23

EXERCISE 5

In order to sit properly you must learn *how to make a lordosis* in the low back while sitting; and then *how to keep a lordosis* in the low back while sitting for prolonged periods. It may take up to eight days of practice to master the correct sitting posture.

How to make a lordosis

Sit on a stool or bench of chair height, or sit sideways on a kitchen chair; allow yourself to slouch completely (photo 33); after having relaxed for a few seconds in the slouched position draw yourself up and accentuate the lordosis (photo 34); after holding the correct position for a few seconds allow yourself to sink back to the slouched position (photo 33). This movement from the slouched to the upright sitting position should be done in such a way that you move rhythmically from the extreme of the 'bad' position to the extreme of the 'good' position. The exercise must be repeated fifteen to twenty times per session, and this must be done three times a day, preferably morning, noon and evening.

It is very important that the movements are done to the extreme ends of your range. In most cases the symptoms will be worst in the extreme slouched position, and much better (or non-existent) in the extreme correct sitting position. In the extreme of the good position there is an increased strain and this may cause pain, often felt in the center of the back, and quite different from your usual low back pain. *Do not be put off by this strain pain:* it should normally occur and will wear off in a few days.

How to keep a lordosis

You have just learned how to find the extreme of the good sitting position (photo 34). It is not possible to sit for long periods in this way as it is a position of strain. If you want to sit comfortably and correctly

24

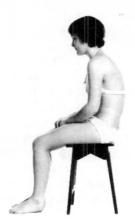

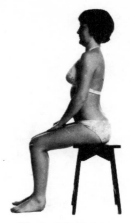

Photo 33: Slouch.

Photo 34: Extreme "good" position.

you must sit just short of the extreme correct position. To find this position, first sit with your back in extreme lordosis (photo 34), and then release the last ten percent of the lordosis strain (photo 35). This position can be maintained comfortably for any length of time. *It is your correct sitting position.*

When sitting like this you keep the lordosis in the low back with your own muscular effort. To effectively hold this position you must constantly pay attention and cannot relax fully. You must sit this way when sitting on a seat *without a back rest.*

When sitting on a chair *with a back rest* you should insert a lumbar support in the small of your back. This enables you to sit relaxed and comfortably, without losing the lordosis. The supportive roll will be discussed later.

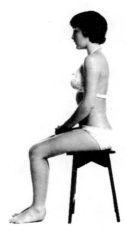

Photo 35: Like 34, but less extreme. This is your correct sitting position.

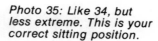

EXERCISE 6

Lie on your back with the knees bent up and your feet flat on the floor or bed (photo 36); draw both knees to your chest (photo 37); place both hands around your knees and pull them firmly but not suddenly against your chest (photo 38); then lower your legs and return to the starting position (do not straighten your knees while lowering your legs). The exercise should be repeated ten times per session, and the sessions should be spread evenly six to eight times throughout the day.

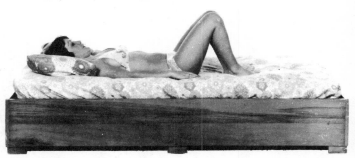

Photo 36

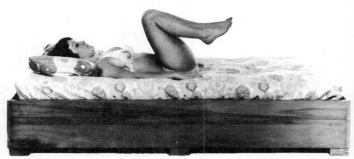

Photo 37

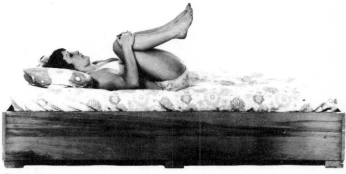

Photo 38

ADVICE AND COMMENTS

Do not continue with any of the exercises if your symptoms are much worse *immediately after exercising* and if they *remain* worse the next day. If any exercise produces or increases leg pain below the knee you should stop it. In either case consult a manipulative therapist.

It is normal to experience some increase in pain or 'new pains' when starting with any new exercises. The new pains are often felt in the arms, up along the back, or between the shoulder blades. They are a sign that the body is performing activities or assuming positions it is not used to. These new pains will diminish as your body gets used to the exercises and they should wear off in a few days.

When you start this exercise programme you should stop any other exercises that you might have been shown elsewhere, or that you happen to do regularly — for example, for fitness or sport. If you want to continue with exercises other than the six given in the last few pages wait until your pains have subsided before doing so.

4

WHEN TO APPLY THE EXERCISES

WHEN YOU ARE IN SIGNIFICANT PAIN
If the pain is very severe, and standing up and walking makes it worse, you should rest in bed and contact your doctor. You must not start with the exercises until you can comfortably lie face down.

If the pain is significant but you are able to walk — you should do Exercises 1 through to 4. Initially you should experience and tolerate some minor increase in pain, but with the repetition of Exercise 3 your back pain should gradually reduce so that there is significant improvement by the time you have done ten movements (or at least after you have finished a few sessions). The pain may also become more localised in the center of the back. *This is desirable,* as is any change of pain *from* the buttocks and legs *towards* the middle of the back. In the end the pain should disappear and be replaced by a feeling of strain and stiffness.

Once you feel considerably better — for example, a day or two after you started with the exercises — you can leave out Exercises 1 and 2, *and as you do this you must start Exercise 5.*

The aim of this part of the programme is first to restore the lordosis and then to maintain it just short of its maximum. As a rule the pain will decrease as your lodosis increases, and you will have no pain once you can obtain the maximum lordosis, but the pain will readily recur as soon as you forget and lose that vital hollow in the small of your back. However, if you maintain the lordosis for some days healing will take place and you will become completely painfree, even when you accidentally lose the lordosis. You will then be able to resume your normal activities. If you follow the instructions given in this book you may also be able to prevent further low back trouble.

WHEN YOU HAVE BEEN PAINFREE FOR TWO TO THREE WEEKS BUT STILL HAVE STIFFNESS ON BENDING FORWARDS
Up till now you have been doing Exercises 1 to 5. While the tissues supporting the spine have healed by maintaining the lordosis for some days, they may also have become less flexible and have shortened as a result of not bending forwards or rounding the back. Therefore, you must now restore the ability to bend forwards without damaging the spine — that is, without tearing the recently healed surfaces.

The risks of further damage to the spine are small when the low back is rounded in a non-weight-bearing position (as in lying), but they become much greater when forward bending is done during weight bearing (as in standing). Exercise 6 allows the low back to become rounded in a non-weight-bearing position.

Exercise 6 should be performed following recovery from an acute episode of low back pain. You should start the exercise when (1) you have been pain free for about two weeks, or (2) you have improved significantly with Exercises 1 to 5, and after two to three weeks are left with a small amount of pain in the center of the back, which does not seem to reduce.

Exercise 6 must *always* be followed by Exercise 3 — that is, ten press-ups while lying face down. In this way you restore the flexibility of your spine in the directions of forward bending as well as backward bending. It also ensures that, after exercising, the discs are placed in the best mechanical position and the vertebrae are lined up properly.

It is not uncommon for some pain to be produced when starting with Exercise 6. An initial pain which wears off gradually with repetition of the exercise is acceptable. It means that shortened tissues are effectively being stretched. However, if Exercise 6 produces pain which increases with each repetition you should stop. In this case it is either too soon to start this phase, or the exercise is not suitable for your condition.

When the knees can touch your chest easily and without discomfort you have regained full movement. Now you can stop Exercise 6, and reduce the programme to that described in the following paragraphs.

WHEN YOU HAVE NO PAIN AND NO STIFFNESS ON BENDING FORWARDS

Let us assume that, like so many people with low back problems, you have lengthy spells when you suffer little or no pain. Even if at the moment you are free of pain, you should start this exercise programme.

You should do Exercises 1 through to 5. After a few days you can adopt a reduced programme, leaving out Exercises 1, 2, and 5, and keeping only Exercises 3 and 4.

In the beginning you must do Exercise 3 before getting up in the morning, repeat it six to eight times per day, and do the last session just before going to bed. After two weeks you may reduce Exercise 3 to twice per day, preferably in the morning and evening; and during the day you may replace Exercise 3 with Exercise 4 whenever it is felt necessary.

In the beginning you must do Exercise 5 three times per day, preferably morning, noon and evening; this may be reduced to once per day after the first week and stopped after two weeks, provided you can achieve and maintain the correct sitting posture, with a good lordosis in the small of your back.

You must be aware of two important points when starting with the programme *while you are pain free.* The first is that you will almost certainly experience new pains; these may be felt in the low back, higher in the back, in shoulders, arms and chest. Be assured that new pains *should* occur when doing new exercises, and they will wear off after a week of practise.

The second point is that, without pain to remind you, you might forget the good sitting posture more easily than people who have pain to remind them as soon as they lose the lordosis. If you do not make a habit of sitting correctly you will have continuing problems and almost certainly suffer another attack of low back pain.

If in the past you have had recurrent episodes of low back pain you should continue with the exercise programme and adopt it as a regular part of your life. It will include: Exercise 3 — twice per day; Exercise 4 — whenever felt necessary; and possibly Exercise 5 — when becoming negligent about the good sitting posture. You must continue with these exercises, even though you are completely pain free at present, in order to prevent future episodes of low back pain. *It may be necessary to exercise in this manner for the rest of your life.*

REMEMBER: *it takes only one minute to perform Exercise 3 ten times; and only two minutes to perform Exercise 5 twenty times.*

5

GENERAL INSTRUCTIONS

1. WHEN YOU ARE IN ACUTE LOW BACK PAIN

You must retain the lordosis at all times. Bending forwards as in touching the toes will only stretch and weaken the supporting structures of the back and lead to further injury. Losing the lordosis when sitting will also cause further strain, and, probably make matters worse.

SITTING
* When in acute pain you should sit as little as possible, and then for short periods only. If you must sit, make sure you have an adequate lordosis. To get this you must place a supportive roll in the small of your back, especially when you are sitting in a car or lounge chair.
* If you have the choice, sit on a firm high chair with a straight back, like a kitchen chair. You should avoid sitting on a low, soft couch with a deep seat which forces you to sit with hips lower than knees, rounded back, and lost lordosis.
* The legs must never be kept straight out in front as in sitting up in bed, or in the bath; in this position you are forced to lose the lordosis in your back.
* When getting up from sitting you must retain the lordosis: Move to the front of the seat, stand up by straightening the legs, and avoid bending forwards at the waist.
* Poor slouched sitting postures are certain to keep you in pain or make you worse.

DRIVING A CAR
* When in acute pain you should drive the car as little as possible, It is better to be a passenger than to drive yourself.
* When driving, your seat must be close enough to the steering wheel to allow you to maintain the lordosis. If in this position your hips are lower than your knees you may be able to raise yourself by sitting on a pillow.

BENDING FORWARDS
* When in acute pain you should avoid activities which require bending forwards or stooping, as these will force you to lose the lordosis.
* You may be able to retain the lordosis by kneeling or going down on all fours when making the bed, vacuuming, cleaning the floor, or weeding the garden.

LIFTING
* When you are in acute pain, avoid lifting.
* If you must lift you should not lift objects that are awkward or heavier than about thirty pounds.
* Always use the correct lifting technique: during lifting the back must remain upright and not stooped or bent forward; stand close to the load, have a firm footing and wide stance; bend the knees to go down to the load and keep the back straight; get a secure grip on the load; lift by straightening the knees; take a steady lift and do not jerk; shift your feet to turn so that you do not twist your back.

LYING
* A good firm support is usually desirable when lying. If your bed sags, slats or plywood supports between mattress and base will firm it. Perhaps someone else can put your mattress on the floor, and you can sleep on it there for a few days.
* You may be more comfortable at night when you

wear a supportive roll. A rolled up towel, wound around your waist and tied in front, is usually satisfactory.
* When getting up from lying you must retain the lordosis; turn on one side, draw both knees up and drop the feet over the edge of the bed; sit up straight by pushing yourself up with your hands, and avoid bending forwards at the waist.

COUGHING AND SNEEZING
* When in acute pain you must try to stand up, bend backwards and increase the lordosis *while* you cough and sneeze.

REMEMBER
* *At all times* you must retain the lordosis; if you slouch you will have discomfort and pain.
Good posture is the key to spinal comfort.

2. WHEN YOU HAVE RECOVERED FROM ACUTE LOW BACK PAIN

You have recovered from the acute episode because you have mastered the exercises which relieved your pain. You can use the same exercises to prevent a recurrence of low back pain, but it is essential that you do them *before the onset of pain*.

If you carry out the following instructions, you can resume normal life without the fear of recurrence.

SITTING
* When sitting for prolonged periods the maintenance of the lordosis is essential. It does not matter if you maintain this with your own muscles or with the help of a supportive roll, placed in the small of your back.
* In addition to sitting correctly with a lumbar support, you should interrupt prolonged sitting at regular intervals. On extended car journeys you should get out of the car every hour or two, stand upright, bend backwards five or six times, and walk around for a few minutes.

BENDING FORWARDS
* When engaged in activities that entail prolonged forward bending or stooping — for example, gardening, vacuuming, concreting — you must

regularly stand upright, restore the lordosis and bend backwards five or six times *before pain commences.*

* Frequent interruption of prolonged forward bending by straightening up and bending backwards to restore and accentuate the lordosis should enable you to continue with most of the activities you are used to doing.

LIFTING
* If the load to be lifted weighs over thirty pounds, the strain must be taken with the low back in lordosis and your knees bent. You must lift by straightening your legs.
* If the object weighs under thirty pounds less care is required, unless you have been in a bent or sitting position for some time prior to lifting. If this has happened you must lift as though the weight exceeds thirty pounds.
* In addition to correct lifting technique, you must stand upright and bend backwards five or six times before and after lifting.

RECURRENCE
* At the first signs of recurrence of low back pain you should immediately start the exercises which previously led to recovery, and follow the instructions given to relieve acute pain.
* If this episode of low back pain seems to be different from previous occasions, and if your pain persists despite your close following of the instructions, you should contact a manipulative therapist.

REMEMBER:
If you lose the lordosis for any length of time, you are risking recurrence of low back pain.

SUMMARY

If you follow the programme carefully and as directed you will benefit in three ways:

1. *You will be painfree while sitting.*
Sitting is the most troublesome position for patients with low back pain.

The exercises will enable you to restore the lost movement in your low back that prevented you from sitting correctly, and you will learn how to sit with an adequate lordosis.

2. *You will be able to treat your low back pain yourself.*
If you have inadvertently stooped or slouched for too long, and have low back pain as a result, you must at once start Exercise 3 — press-ups —; or, if this is not possible, Exercise 4 — bending backwards while standing. Regain your lordosis slowly and carefully, never suddenly or jerkily, for a little time is required for the distorted discs to regain their normal shape. A sudden and violent movement may overhasten this process and cause strain in and around the discs, with an increase of low back pain.

What has happened is that you have taught yourself how to 'put your back in', after having discovered painfully the various ways in which you may 'put your back out'. The simple rule is that if bending forwards 'puts the back out', bending backwards will 'put it back in'.

3. *You will be able to prevent further attacks of low back pain.*
If you interrupt prolonged bending and stooping *before pain starts* by applying Exercise 3 or Exercise 4 to restore and accentuate the lordosis, you will not 'put your back out'.

YOUR DIARY: Low back attacks or episodes

Date Be sure to include the year.	How much pain? 1 (low) to 5 (high) scale Where? Use photos on page 9 as reference.	What caused the episode?	Did y profe help?

My name and address (optional)_____

you fill in this table you are
ing valuable research data, I'd be
ful if you would photo copy it, and send it to me.

POST TO: Robin McKenzie
Physiotherapy Clinic, Kelvin Chambers
16 The Terrace, Wellington, New Zealand

What exercises did you do? per 1, 2, 3, 4, 5, 6 as on pages 21-26.) What else did you do?	How long did this episode last? What benefit did you get from the advice contained in this book?

SUMMARY
Has advice from this book speeded your   YES
recovery from episodes of low back pain? NO

Has it helped you to avoid episodes?   YES
                                           NO